MY JOURNEY TO GUINNESS

MY JOURNEY TO GUINNESS

"WALKING DIVA" WALKING MY WAY INTO THE
GUINNESS BOOK OF WORLD RECORDS

YOLANDA HOLDER

authorHOUSE®

AuthorHouse™
1663 Liberty Drive
Bloomington, IN 47403
www.authorhouse.com
Phone: 1-800-839-8640

Published by AuthorHouse   03/26/2012

ISBN: 978-1-4685-6280-4 (sc)
ISBN: 978-1-4685-6279-8 (e)

Library of Congress Control Number: 2012904574

Any people depicted in stock imagery provided by Thinkstock are models, and such images are being used for illustrative purposes only.
Certain stock imagery © Thinkstock.

This book is printed on acid-free paper.

Because of the dynamic nature of the Internet, any web addresses or links contained in this book may have changed since publication and may no longer be valid. The views expressed in this work are solely those of the author and do not necessarily reflect the views of the publisher, and the publisher hereby disclaims any responsibility for them.

CONTENTS

DEDICATION

God grant me the Serenity
To accept the things I cannot change
Courage to change the things I can and
Wisdom to know the difference
-Serenity Prayer-

The Diving Board

This book is dedicated to my father James Wesley Hampton who passed away July 7, 2003. My father who we called "Jimmy" was a recovering alcoholic who believed in the Twelve Step Program. My fondest memory at the age of ten was when he took me and a few of my other sibling swimming at the YMCA. I had learned to jump off the edge of the pool into the deep end which was 8 or 10 feet. Each jump I screamed with joy "Jimmy watch". After about three or four times jumping off the edge, Jimmy said, "Jump off the diving board". I looked at him with fear in my eyes and replied okay. As I climbed up the ladder, which was only three steps, fear set in and my heart began to pound. I walked to the end of the diving board and looked down, I wanted to turn and run back. I looked over at Jimmy and he said "jump, you will come up to the top and swim to me." The line for the diving board was getting long, but the kids were patient because they knew this was my first jump off the diving board. Jimmy said to me, "trust me you can do it, jump!" Finally after what felt like hours standing there I jumped, floated to the top and swam to Jimmy. He replied, "The first jump is always the hardest." As the years went by and I ran into scary or unsettling situations, Jimmy would always remind me of the "Diving Board". This was one of those life lessons that stayed with me. My journey to Guinness had a lot of bumps in the road but Jimmy was with me every step of the way. When fear got in the way, the Diving Board always came to mind.

ACKNOWLEDGMENTS

To thank everyone who has helped me on my journey would be impossible. There is however key people that played significant roles in my life that I would like to acknowledge.

First I would like to thank my husband Roger. He has always believed in me and has supported me with his love and encouragement. I love you!

Huge thanks goes to my wonderful son RJ for his professional advice and editing skills. You pushing me gave me the courage to write this book. Thank you and I love you.

To my sweet daughter Tiffany who I love and admire so much. Thanks for listening to my endless venting. Your prayers and strong belief in God is what got me through the tough times. You are my love, my heart, and the best daughter I could ask for.

Thank you to my mother for your words of wisdom—"Don't let anyone steal your joy!"

Girlfriends are forever! To Cheryl Arnold, Veronica Richason and Angela Summers, each one of you played a very special role in my journey and words just can't explain how grateful and blessed I am to have each of you in my life.

Thank you to my marathon walking buddy MG Montgomery for keeping me grounded and laughing. A special thank you to my marathon friend Irlan Hebner and good friend Debbie Myers for endless conversations and words of encouragement.

A special thank you goes to Shannon Jones for her editing skills and selflessness. God sent me an Angel and I would not have gotten this book finished if it wasn't for you.

Most importantly I thank God for giving me the courage to step out of my comfort zone and believe in myself to become the amazing woman that I am today.

To understand my journey to Guinness, you must understand my past. I grew up in a blended family with the malefactor effects of alcoholism and abuse. Both my mother and father had three children from a previous marriage, they fell in love and once married had eight additional children. Growing up one of fourteen children wasn't easy. Being the middle child can be confusing and as a result I suffered the perils of middle child syndrome—namely, feeling not sure where I fit in. My father who I loved dearly suffered from alcoholism. He later was able to free himself of his addiction when I was five, through hard work and the positive reinforcement of the Twelve Step Program. The Twelve Step Program did not only impact my father's life but mine as well. Each step has symbolically played a role in my journey to becoming a Guinness World Record holder. My father's passion shows me that believing in my dreams and having the desire to motivate and help others reach their goal was a rewarding feeling.

In 2003 my father passed away due to diabetes complications. My father battled fifteen years of diabetes that caused many complications that included three triple by passes, a leg amputation and loss of sight. His brave and courageous spirit lives on each time I cross a finish line.

CHAPTER ONE

WHAT'S MY MOTIVATION?

2007 was definitely a life changing year for me. It was the year marathons went from being a hobby to my passion. I was never athletic growing up. I belonged to my local gym and would take step aerobics classes when I could find time from my full time job as a devoted wife and mother of two. It wasn't until I turned forty when I started to walk and occasionally participate in local marathons.

May 2007 at the Rock N Roll San Diego Marathon I spotted a gentleman wearing a shirt that read "Fifty States Marathon Club", a club were the members share a common goal of completing a marathon in all fifty states. I immediately knew this was something I needed to be a part of. To join, a runner must have completed a marathon in at least ten states. I had already completed in four different states, "This was an achievable goal", I thought to myself, and so I set out to be a member of the Fifty States Club. While pursuing membership with the Fifty States Club, I saw a group of men at the San Francisco Marathon wearing these bright yellow singlets that said "Marathon Maniacs" and I knew I had to have one. The easiest way to join the Marathon Maniacs was to run three marathons in ninety days. In September of 2007, I joined the "Maniac" family, where I picked up the nick name "Walking Diva".

In November of 2007 I was set to complete my tenth race in the Seattle Marathon. The completion of this race was both exciting and bittersweet. I had reached my goal in order to become a Fifty States Club member, but what next? Marathon's had quickly become more than just a way to stay fit; they brought a sense of fulfillment to my life and helped me to find peace within. Marathons had also brought a great new group of friends in my life that shared the same interests and goals as I did; I knew the marathon community had more in store for me.

The morning of the Seattle Marathon I ran into my marathon friend Todd "Barefoot Runner" Byers. We spoke about how my fiftieth birthday was soon approaching and how I wanted to do something fun and exciting to celebrate such a milestone in my life. I was ending a chapter in my life, my forties, and starting a new chapter, my fifties. I decided in that moment I would complete fifty marathons in fifty-two weeks. To my surprise Todd said, "Yolanda, I have no doubt that you can do this". I left the Seattle Marathon with a new goal and more motivated than ever!

In order to complete my goal I participated in a combination of different marathons: road marathons, ultra marathons, and trail marathons. Before I became familiar with trail marathons, I had a challenging experience at the Napa Valley Trail Marathon. It was my first and I had no idea what was in store for me. It was an uphill trail with no mile markers, just orange ribbons to guide participants in the right direction. I ran through creeks, climbed over fallen trees, hopped over rocks, fell in the dirt and got lost. As I made my way back to the finish line, I said, "Never again will I do a trail marathon". Later that day I reflected on the challenges I endured while at the marathon and realized how connected I was with God.

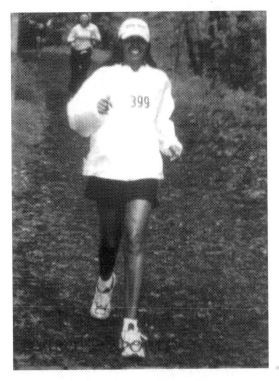

Napa Valley Trail Marathon

Trail marathons quickly became my favorite to participate in. They were both challenging and beautiful at the same time. I participated in the Golden Gate Headlands Trail Marathon the following week. I was so motivated to complete my goal I began doing double marathons and even triple marathons. I was fifty years young and amazed at what my body was doing!

October, 26, 2008, I finished my fiftieth marathon of the year at the Silicon Valley Marathon. I was excited and couldn't believe that I was ahead of schedule. I still had eight weeks left in the year. I stayed committed to my decision, but stayed flexible in my approach and reached my goal. I was learning to trust myself, and allowed the strong fearless woman within me to shine.

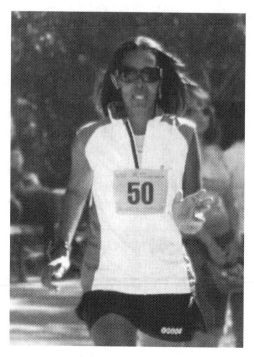

Silicon Valley Marathon

We all have different platforms in life and mine was power walking marathons. I completed my first triple marathon, the Lake Tahoe Triple. The triple consists of three different marathons in three days in two states. The event covers the entire shoreline of beautiful Lake Tahoe over three days for a total of 78.6 miles! The highlight of 2008 was finishing the JFK fifty miler in 13:03:48 and completing the Philadelphia Marathon in 6:14:34 that following day. I finished 2008 surpassing my original goal of fifty marathons in fifty-two weeks. Instead I completed sixty-five marathons which included a triple marathon and a fifty miler. To round out an already awesome year I was awarded 2008 Marathon Maniac of the Year and Vasque Envirosports 2008 Queen of the Mountain Champion.

After power walking sixty-five marathons in one year, I felt invincible. I was on cloud nine and decided I would try out for the show Wipe Out. I went on the show website and emailed them, the producer called, and a few weeks later I was on the show. I wiped out on every single event. My episode was food and I faced the banana split, onion rings, and the motivator. All three obstacle courses sent me flying, crashing and banged me up pretty bad. The only thing I left with was an injured back and battered body. With a hurt back and all I continued to power walk marathons.

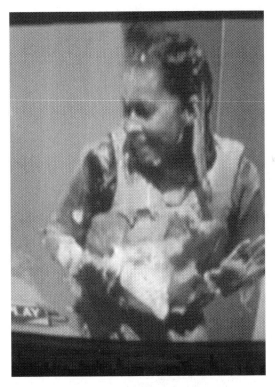

Wipeout

Chapter Two

2009

In 2009 I went on to walk seventy-seven marathons. One of my favorite marathons was the Goofy Challenge at Walt Disney World. I love bling (medals) and the Disney Corporation awards some of the most beautiful medals. The Goofy Challenge is a 39.3 mile adventure held over two days. Saturday is the Donald Duck half marathon and Sunday the Mickey Mouse marathon. If you finish both races within the time limits you are awarded the coveted Goofy medal in addition to your Donald Duck and Mickey Mouse finisher medals.

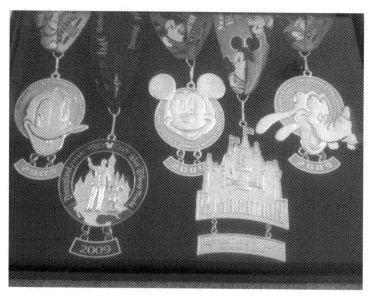

Coast to coast Walt Disney Medals

I did the Disneyland Half Marathon so that I could own the Coast to Coast medal. If you complete the Disneyland half in California and a marathon or half in Walt Disney World in the same calendar year, you are awarded the coast to coast medal. I enjoyed walking through the parks and taking pictures with the celebrities. I had a magical time at both races!

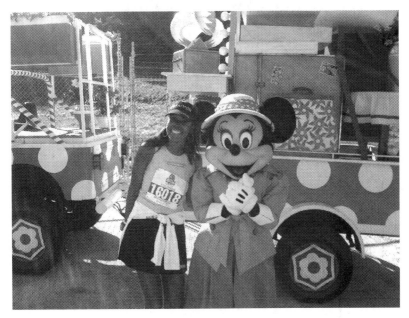

Goofy Challenge

Twenty—seven of the seventy-seven marathons I completed were ultra marathons. If a road marathon wasn't available then I would power walk a 50k. I power walked some of the most beautiful trails in California. These trails were very challenging but beautiful, with spectacular views of the Pacific Ocean and city views. I found serenity on the trails. The peace and calm during the races became therapeutic and encouraged me to move forward in the hopes to see more of what nature's beauty had to show me.

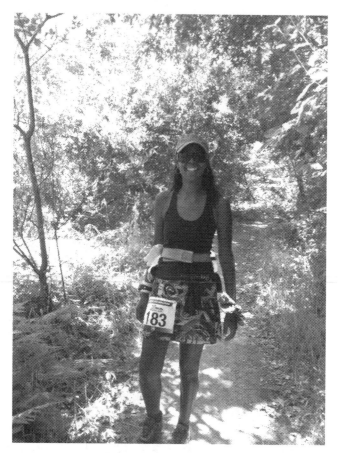

Skyline 50K

One of the toughest trail marathons was Leadville Marathon in Colorado. The course toured the historic mining district on the East side of Leadville, reaching elevation heights of 13,000 feet at Mosquito Pass. The altitude and mosquitoes were working against me that day. At the aid station at mile twenty-two the volunteer said "Good bye and I will see you again in an hour or so". As she pointed up to the mountain, I realized I would have to walk up and around the tumultuous peak. I looked at her in disbelief and began to cry. I later learned that low sugar levels in women have symptoms such as crying.

I had topped my previous year's record in marathons and became once again, Marathon Maniac of the Year 2009 and Pacific Coast Trail Champion 2009. I was itching for a new challenge, so I checked with Guinness to see who was holding the title of "Most Marathons Run in a Calendar Year" by a woman. I knew I could break the record, so I entered the new year with a new goal in mind, the Guinness World Record!

Chapter Three

JANUARY 2010

I did ten marathons in January of 2010. My schedule for 2010 was packed with doubles and triple marathons. I was still tired from seventy-seven marathons the previous year and sixty-five marathons in 2008, but extremely excited to take on my new challenge of one hundred and one marathons for the Guinness World Record!

I started off setting a personal best of 5:26:57, in my first marathon of the year at the Texas Marathon in Kingswood. Marathon's three and four were both in Southern states. At the Mississippi Blues Marathon in Jackson, I was welcomed with cold weather that literally turned me blue! My hands and toes were frozen which made it hard to walk. It took a twenty minute shower to finally thaw me out. What got me through the cold was what was waiting for me at the finish line, an awesome finisher's medal! I finished 6:02:51.

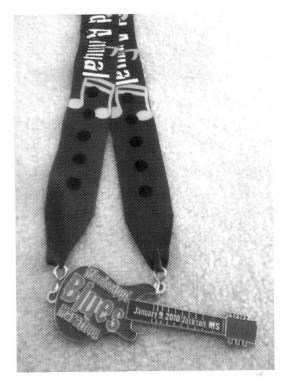

Mississippi Blues medal

The drive to Mobile was a three and a half hour drive from Jackson. First Light Marathon was just as cold as the Mississippi Blues Marathon. I couldn't wait to get back home to sunny California. I finished in 6:09:49.

On January 15th I drove from California to Phoenix to pick up my race packet for the Rock N Roll Arizona Marathon taking place in just two days. In order to maintain momentum in breaking the Guinness Record I couldn't allow too many unproductive days. I had my son RJ drop me off at the Phoenix Airport where I flew to Atlanta for the Museum of Aviation Marathon, in Warner Robins Georgia. It rained the whole marathon. I finished wet and cold in 5:42:48. I arrived in Phoenix and my son picked me up and I spent the night with him. The start of the Rock N Roll Arizona Marathon was cold but quickly warmed up to a nice seventy degrees. It felt so good to be on the West Coast where the weather is dry and warm! My legs were sore but I did manage to pull off a strong finish of 5:49:05.

Marathon number seven was supposed to be Diamond Valley Lake Marathon but was canceled due to flooding. I received the message on Friday afternoon of the cancellation so I immediately checked the web to find another race. Yuma Marathon in Arizona was the closest marathon. I drove all night and arrived at 5:30am and the marathon started at 7am. I finished in 5:40:33. The drive home was long and exhausting, I Arrived home only to have to wake up by three a.m. the following morning.

I set a goal for myself to try and finish my marathons under six hours. The start of marathon number eight, the Carlsbad Marathon was cold and in the low thirties. The Carlsbad course is beautiful with miles of ocean views. I finished in 5:56:16. Marathon number nine was the Desert Classic Marathon in Arizona and being so busy, I forgot to buy my airline tickets. Always have a plan B! I drove to Arizona and stayed with my son. I started early so that I wouldn't have any problems making my 2:55 fight to Dallas. I finished in 5:54:17 and made my flight!

My final marathon of the month was Miracle Match Marathon in Waco, Texas. This marathon was very special to me. Waco Texas is where my father was born; he would tell me stories about Waco quite often. The course was nice and scenic. I was feeling ill but imagining my father enjoying the land and fresh air as he would often recollect, kept me motivated to finish the race. I started to feel worse as the day went on. By the time I finished, my chest was burning and I was losing my voice. The next morning I felt so bad that I went to the doctor and was diagnosed with bronchitis. It was all worth it! I was able to feel my father's presence all 6:03:49 of the race. I know it was him that got me to the finish line.

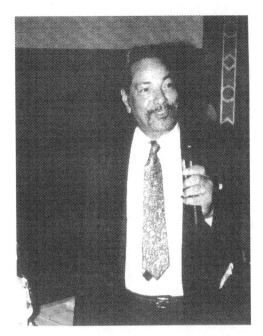

My father Jimmy

Chapter Four

FEBRUARY 2010

My first race in February was Diamond Valley Lake Marathon, in Hemet, California and I was happy that I didn't have to travel that weekend. It was canceled the previous month due to flooding and rescheduled, but once again the weather was awful. It rained so hard the first half, the race director called the race off. After much persuasion he let a few of us continue on. It was wet, cold and muddy, but by the second half the rain stopped and I finished in 6:26:46.

Marathon number twelve was the Surf City Marathon, California Dreaming Series and this was my 3rd year completing the series. If you complete a marathon or half at San Francisco Marathon, Long Beach Marathon and Surf City Marathon in the same calendar year you receive a beautiful medal.

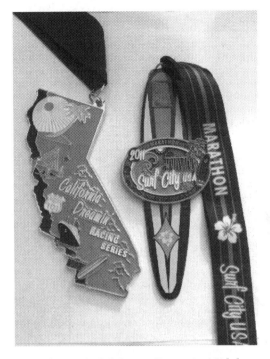

Surf City & California Dreamin medals

The following weekend was a triple marathon holiday weekend. Holidays are perfect for participating in triple marathons. Pemberton Trail 50k was my first 50k and triple of the year. The Pemberton 50K is run on trails in the beautiful McDowell Mountain Regional Park in Scottsdale Arizona; it has rolling hills and two loops which we had to finish within 4 hours each. Lost Dutchman Marathon was my fourteenth marathon of the year. It was filled with nice and friendly people, always a plus when participating in marathons. We were bused to the start at Peralta Trailhead and welcomed with campfires to keep us warm. Six miles of the course was scenic with rolling hills on unpaved roads with beautiful desert vistas, there were also awesome views of the famous superstition Mountains. I finished in 5:58:41 and immediately drove home to California.

Day three of my triple was Love your Heart Marathon, held at Central Park in Huntington Beach California. It was not only beautiful but heart-warming, because my younger sister Stacy accompanied me. She's a runner and had not run a marathon in a while, but she wasn't going to let her older sister beat her while power walking. Power Walking is an underrated technique that gets overlooked in the marathon world. For me it was a new and exciting way to stay fit without becoming vulnerable to certain health risks that are associated with running. Stacy finished 6:29:03 and I finished 6:31:06 and not to mention that was my third marathon in three days!

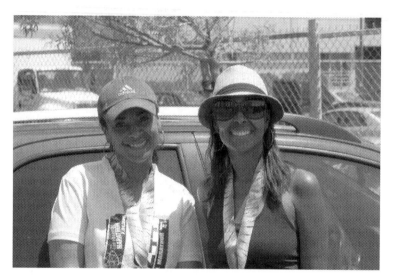

My sister Stacy and I

Marathon number sixteen was the Orange Curtain 50K in Cerritos California which meant I didn't have to travel to get there and was able to sleep in. The Orange Curtain 50K is an out and back run along the bike path of the San Gabriel River. I met the legendary Jim Simpson who has run over seven hundred lifetime marathons and I had the pleasure of walking with him. I finished in 7:39:32. To finish off my no travel weekend I participated in the Pasadena Marathon and once again race day was the object of Mother Nature's mischief; chilly rain in the morning and sunshine in the afternoon. I loved the scenic course and ran around the famous Pasadena Rose Bowl. I finished in 6:22:37.

I'm rested and ready for what I call a fast weekend. Marathon number eighteen was the Cowtown Marathon in Ft. Worth, Texas. At this point I had gotten used to the weather being in the low forties. Cowtown Marathon was a friendly marathon that starts and finishes in the Will Rogers Memorial Center, the heart of the cultural district in Fort Worth. I finished in 5:57:42. I flew from Dallas to New Orleans for the Inaugural Mardi Gras Rock N Roll Marathon. This was my nineteenth marathon for the year and my first time in New Orleans. Secretly I was more excited about having gumbo and beignets than actually walking the marathon. One of the great things about doing marathons is that you get to travel to places that you've never been. New Orleans was one of those places I've heard so much about and wanted to visit. The marathon course toured the French Quarter and Bourbon Street, scenic and majestic St., Charles Avenue, the stately Garden District and two of the loveliest urban parks—Audubon Park and City Park. I finished in 6:04:35 and off I went to have my gumbo and beignets, what a treat! The Mardi Gras Rock N Roll Marathon became very special to me. I met the most amazing person, Tony "Endorphin Dude". Tony has an amazing story and marathoning has changed his life forever. I finished nine marathons in February and was on a role!

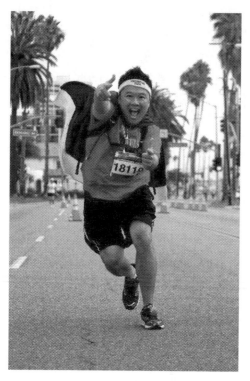

Tony "Endorphin Dude"

CHAPTER FIVE

MARCH 2010

Marathon number twenty was the Red Rock Canyon Marathon in Las Vegas. I live three hours away so I chose to drive, which meant I had to leave at 2 am. We were bused to the start and it was very cold, in the low forties. The marathon course is an out and back route on a paved road that winds through the Red Rock Canyon National Conservation Area with a climb of 4,771 feet. There was a breathtaking scenic overlook view of the ruddy sandstone cliffs, cacti and Joshua trees. I finished in 6:03:43 and drove straight home.

I got up at 3am the following morning feeling tired and sore. Marathon twenty one was Malibu Creek Trail 50k in Malibu, California. The weather was cold and overcast with an 8.5 hour cutoff. The course is located in the Santa Monica Mountains with river crossings, spectacular views of the ocean and a gain of 5,940 feet. The 50K consists of two loops with a four hour cutoff on the first loop. The afternoon views of the ocean are spectacular. I finished 8:23:38.

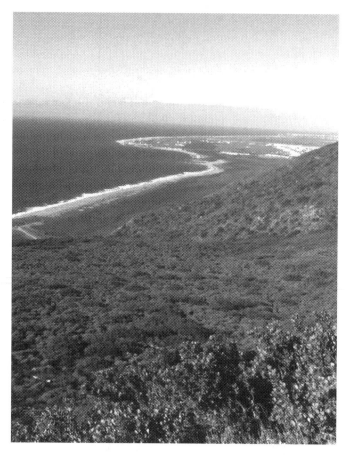

Malibu Creek Trail 50K

Race number twenty-three was the Redwood Park marathon. I did something I had never done; I drove all night and arrived in Oakland, California, an eight hour drive to participate in the marathon, thank goodness for girlfriends! My friend Cheryl and I talked all night until I arrived at the start safely. Redwood Park Trail Marathon is one of my favorite trails; you can really lose yourself in the natural scenery. The course travels through the beautiful Redwood Regional Park and has spectacular views of tall redwoods with streams and French trails. It rained the first six miles which made the trails so wet and muddy, I sprained my right ankle. I went on to do nine marathons on my ankle before my husband insisted I go to the doctor. That was my only injury during my journey. I finished in 6:38:47 and was able to drive myself home.

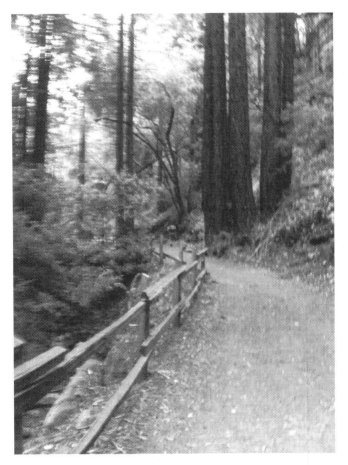

Redwood Park Marathon

Race number twenty—five I got a few hours of sleep and got up excited and ready for one of my favorite marathons, the LA Marathon. I was one fourth of my journey to Guinness! I didn't have to worry about driving because LA marathon is my husband's favorite marathon also, he always drives my marathon buddy Brenda and myself to the race. LA Marathon changed owners and has a new course, I love it! We started at Dodger Stadium and finished in Santa Monica. The course traveled through Hollywood, Beverly Hills, and Rodeo Drive. I finished in 6:32:36 and survived another fast pace weekend!

Races twenty-six and twenty-seven were both in the San Francisco Bay Area which made me extremely happy. Finally I had a weekend with no traveling from one end of the state to the other. Napa Trail Marathon is held in the beautiful Napa Wine Country. This was my third Napa Trail Marathon and I had become familiar with the course. I love the scenery and beautiful silence. At this point I had gotten used to being alone on the trails and not afraid of getting lost. I had a great day and finished in 5:32:58 which was a trail marathon personal record! The Inaugural Oakland Marathon was really nice. The course traveled around the beautiful Lake Merritt, Jack London Square and the historic Claremont Hills.

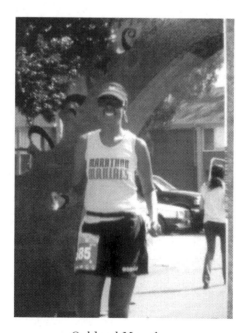

Oakland Marathon

The community came together and supported their city. I was very impressed the way Oakland showcased their diverse neighborhoods. I finished in 6:08:30 and was handed a beautiful medal and zip up t-shirt. I finished the month off with eight marathons.

CHAPTER SIX

APRIL 2010

Doing a marathon is 90% mental and 10% physical. I've learned a lot about myself and I'm determined to break the Guinness World Record. I had to drive all night to Sausalito, CA for marathon twenty-eight the Golden Gate Headland Marathon. This trail marathon has it all; spectacular views of San Francisco, Marin Headland, Golden Gate Bridge, Angel Island and beautiful cityscapes. The course is a combination of single track hiking trails, fire roads, and beach crossings. I finished the race in 5:30:07 and drove back home. I've only had a few hours of sleep. The eight hours drive and tough trail marathon I did the previous day is starting to take a toll on my body. Sycamore Canyon Trail 50K was marathon twenty-nine and my fifteenth consecutive back to back double. I've done Sycamore many times and it gets easier each time, I finished in 7:58:00.

The Labor of Love Marathon series is a two day running festival that offers many races. I did three events. I was very nervous because if I didn't finish in the allotted time I could face a DNF (Did Not Finish). I was feeling good and excited. The weather was great and I did Labor of Love last year so I was familiar with the course. I finished the first marathon with no problem in 6:07:51. I changed chip and bib, made myself a burger and off I went to start the Labor of Love 50 Miler. I was doing well until mile thirty-five when I started to get blisters on both feet. Around 1am I started to lose my balance and delirium started to set in. I finished around 3:30am in 14:10:36. The temperature was in the low thirties and I waited in a volunteer's car until the start of the 50k. I started the Labor of Love 50K at 6am. It was still dark, I had blisters on both feet and I was extremely tired but I managed to find the courage and strength to conquer three events that totaled to 107 miles in 28:48:24.

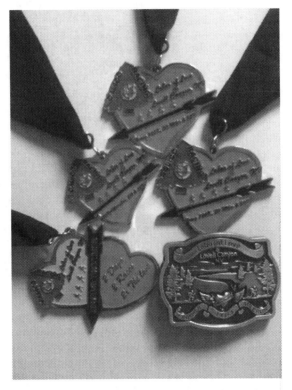

Labor of Love Medals

I made a last minute decision to drive to the Bay Area to participate in the Skyline to the Sea Trail Marathon. I thought I was going to Las Gatos but realized half way into the trip that we were being bused from the finish line in Santa Cruz. I arrived at 2am and took a nap in the car until the buses arrived. This was my first Skyline to the Sea Trail marathon and what a beautiful course. The trail runs from the crest of the Santa Cruz Mountains at Saratoga Gap, through Big Basin Redwoods State Park and ends at the Pacific Ocean. We traveled through tall redwoods, high chaparral and there were many breathtaking waterfalls. I didn't want it to end; I finished in 7:05:16.

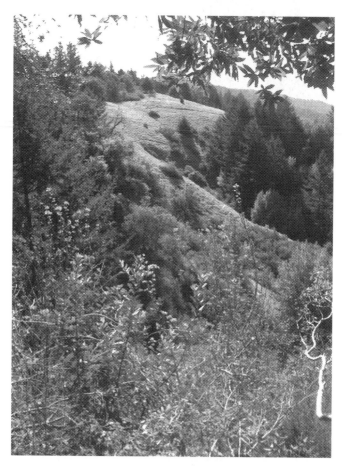

Skyline to the Sea Trail Marathon

The Rocky Road Run Marathon was race number thirty-five. The course was scenic but hard and it reached over 80 degrees by the time I finished. I finished in 6:11:10 and immediately drove to San

Francisco to do race number thirty-six. The Marin County Marathon was an inaugural with a strict cutoff of 6 hours. The course was hilly, and tough but beautiful with spectacular views of the ocean and the mountains. I was born and raised in the Bay Area and being able to see this beautiful city for 26.2 miles was amazing. I met a woman that was our pacer and her amazing story was what started the "amazing person" segment on my blog. With her pacing me I finished in 5:52:50.

CHAPTER SEVEN

MAY 2010

I'm happy that I didn't have to travel back and forth to the Bay Area the first weekend of May. Marathon number thirty-seven was the May Day Madness Trail Marathon. This marathon was on single track trails, with creek crossing in Las Flores, California not far from my home. I like creek crossing especially on hot days. I finished in 6:39:15. The OC Marathon number thirty-eight changed its course this year and we were bused to the start and finished at the OC Fairgrounds. The course had miles of beautiful ocean views; I finished in 5:45:40.

Race number thirty-nine was my first 50K double and fell on my birthday. I spent my birthday at the Quicksilver 50K in San Jose, California. My husband accompanied me which made the marathon that much more exciting. The course was brutal, hilly, challenging and the weather was hot, but seeing my husband at the end of the finish line made it all worth it! I finished in 8:07:48, and received a very nice finisher's medal. What a great birthday it was!

May was my second time this year walking Redwood Park but this time it's a 50K. The trail is one of my favorites. Traveling through the tall redwoods and the awesome views of the surrounding areas is my all time favorite. I did my first double 50K and finished in 8:28:40. What a wonderful birthday weekend!

Palos Verdes Marathon's course is hilly, and challenging but scenic. My body is becoming acclimated to walking back to back double marathons and I'm finding the travel is harder than the actual 26.2 miles. My quads welcome the hills for a change of muscles is helpful. There was a nice site along the course of the famous Trump National Golf Club. I beat last years' time by one minute. I finished in 5:59:16.

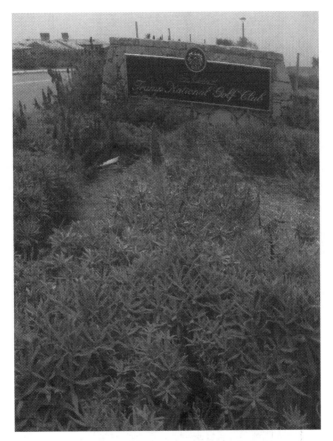

Trump National Golf Club

Going Bananas Marathon number forty-two was held at Legg Lake Park and the course was a 2.2 mile that loops around a fast, flat and scenic lake. The weather was cool at the start but I was feeling tired from the quad workout at the Palos Verdes Marathon. I finished in 6:48:52.

Marathon number forty-three was the Rocky Horror Marathon in Coto De Caza, California. Wow! It sure did live up to its name, the course was BRUTAL! The race director is an ultra—marathoner and was the course designer. The course was hilly with a seven thousand elevation gain. At the start of the trail there was a sign that said, "Beware of mountain lions", it should have read, "Beware of rattle snakes". I spent more time screaming than actually power walking. The trails were not groomed and I saw two snakes. The course was so tough, that I finished in a disappointing 9:18:42.

Nanny Goat 12/24 Hour Race, number forty-five took place on a one mile dirt loop on a private horse ranch located in Riverside, California ten miles from my home. This was Nanny Goats second year and mine also. It's becoming a party with fun runners, good food and excellent swags with a nice goat finisher's medal. This year I opted to do only 32 miles and finished under nine hours.

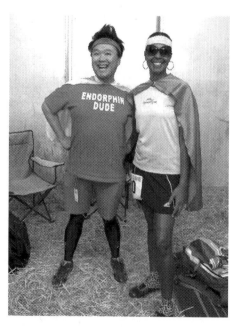

Tony "Endorphin Dude" and the "Walking Diva Dudette"

Memorial Day Weekend Marathon was run on an incredibly scenic bike path in Huntington Beach, California. The course is a 6.5 mile out and back along the beach. It's awesome to see Southern Californians getting out and enjoying life and I specially loved the yoga on the beach. I finished in7:29:09. I finished the month of May with ten marathons.

CHAPTER EIGHT

JUNE 2010

I have done many trails in the Bay Area but never the Diablo Trail 50K. The course was hilly and scenic on single track trails and dirt roads. The 25K course climbs to the summit and the 50K does two loops to the summit. Once you reach the summit it's worth the climb, it was breathtaking and magnificent! On the second loop to the summit I got heat exhaustion but managed to finish in 9:58:11.

June 11, 2010 was a triple marathon weekend. I participated in the Bear Lake Idaho, Bear Lake Marathon and Estes Park Marathon. Three marathons, in three states in, three days! I flew into Salt Lake City and drove two hours to Garden City Idaho. I met up with my friend Roxana and she and I car camped. The weather was freezing and it rained all night. The car was uncomfortable, I didn't sleep a wink. Arriving at the start it was so cold that I thought it was January 11th not June 11th. It rained 90% of the marathon, but I was able to complete it in 6:14:20. Roxana and I met up to take showers but I just couldn't car camp another night, so I drove an hour to Utah and stayed the night in a hotel. Feeling rested and relaxed, I was ready for day two of the triple. The amazing thing about doing a triple is that your body gets faster each day. I managed to shave three minutes off my time from the previous day. I finished in 6:11:09.

My fight into Colorado was delayed due to thunder storms. Although my plane was delayed forty-five minutes, I didn't panic; I arrived in

Estes Park ready to conquer the triple marathon. The weather was wet and cold and it rained for miles and miles. What I have learned over the last three years is that you can't control Mother Nature, so why be miserable for 6 hours when you can embrace the weather with a smile. I finished my third consecutive marathon in 5:55:52. I was half way to the Guinness World Record!

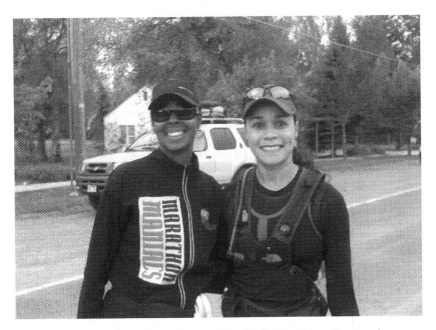

Bear Lake Marathon. Irlan and I, she finished her first triple

I drove all night to San Francisco and arrived in Tiburon around 4am for the Angel Island 50K race number fifty-one. I got a few hours of sleep before the ferry ride to Angel Island. It was a beautiful morning. We got lucky and could not have asked for a more beautiful day in the bay. The course had panoramic views of San Francisco and the trail to the summit was breathtaking, the Island itself has a lot of history. The dreaded stairs almost made me forget about the serine trail. What a quad busters! I finished in7:32:00.

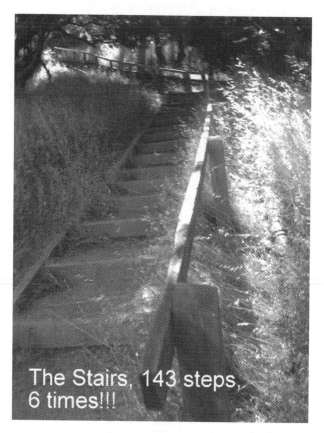

The Stairs, 143 steps, 6 times!!!

Angel Island 50K

The Father's Day Marathon was held on a well groomed horse trail in beautiful Coto de Caza, California. I was feeling excited that my journey to Guinness was possible as long as I stayed positive and focused. I took my time and finished in 7:09:50

Race number fifty-three was my fourth triple of my journey to the Guinness. It wasn't as challenging as the other three because it didn't require as much traveling. Five Cities Coastal Marathon in Oceanside, California travels through five cities: Oceanside, Carlsbad, Leucadia, Encinitas and Cardiff. The race started at the historical Café 101 restaurant in Oceanside, I finished in 6:59:10.

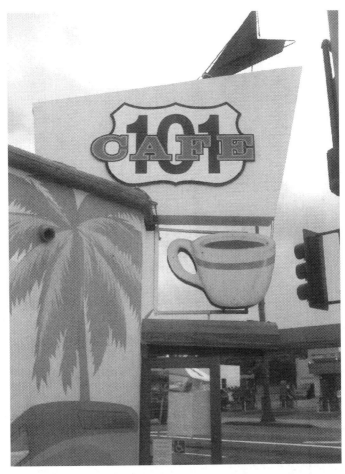

Five Cities Coastal Marathon. Café 101 restaurant.

Marathon number fifty-four was my love to hate race, Running with the Devil Marathon. Its run in over one hundred degree heat, the first year I ran it, it was one hundred and fifteen degrees. This year I got lucky it was only one hundred and five degrees. At the start of the race you're weighed and again at mile thirteen. I started at 7am with fifty milers and was so happy that I was feeling great and didn't lose any weight at the half way point. I spoke too soon, at mile twenty heat exhaustion set in but I did manage to finish in 7:20:34.

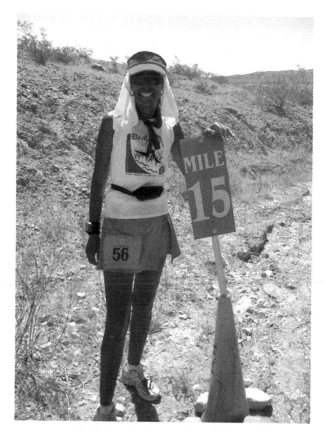

Running with the Devil Marathon

The Running with Todd Marathon, and day three of my triple was held at Legg Lake Park in El Monte, California. Many runners asked me if I was okay because I looked very thin. I explained that I did "Running with the Devil" the previous day and lost a few pounds. The first half of the marathon was nice and cool compared to yesterday, but I must say I wanted this marathon over. I finished in 6:41:17.

CHAPTER NINE

JULY 2010

The Stars and Stripes Marathon was day one of my first back to back triples. I like the marathons that are held on Huntington Beach Pier because of the endless miles of incredibly scenic ocean views. I finished the marathon in 6:18:50. I arrived in Portland, Oregon for the Foot Traffic Flat Marathon number fifty-seven, which was held on the fourth of July. I always get to marathons at least an hour and half before the start and in this marathon I am so glad I did. I got lost and the traffic getting to the start was so bad that runners were getting out of their cars and running to the start. The weather was great and the course was nice with strawberry fields along the course. They served us the best strawberry shortcake at the end of the race. I finished in 6:07:07.

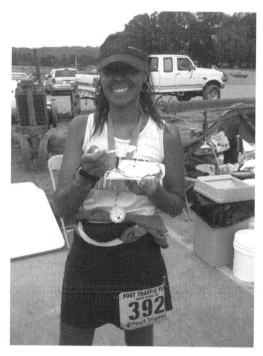

Foot Traffic Flat Marathon

Day three of my triple back to back was the Independence Day Marathon, which was held in beautiful Coto de Caza, CA. I completed my first triple back to back; the impossible was possible after all. The Dirty Dozen 12/6 Hour Endurance Run marathon number fifty-nine was held at Pinole State Park, in Pinole, California. The course was a 3.1 mile loop with pretty views of the ocean. The trail was scenic with nice smelling eucalyptus trees. I managed to finish thirty-two miles in 8:26:25 and won first place in my age group.

I've decided to do something I've never done before. Two trail marathons in one day. Headland Marathon race number sixty-one started at Rodeo Beach in Sausalito, California. I have done these trails many times but this time the race director decided to change the course. It was so cool; I saw wild turkeys and finished the race in 7:15:25.

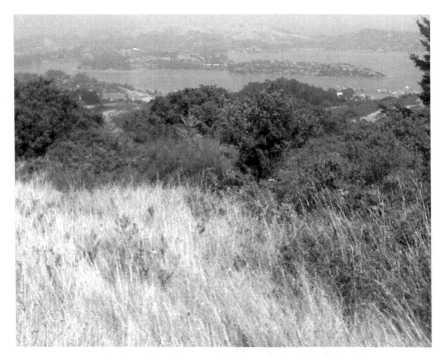

Headland Marathon. Sausalito, California

The drive to Cool Moon 12 Hour Run in Cool, California was a 2.5 hour drive from Sausalito. I arrived to Cool and it was over one hundred degrees, talk about an oxymoron. I started the race at 6pm. I needed to finish three out of nine loops tonight in order to complete the race in time. I'm not a good night walker, and it was so hot that many runners dropped and I knew I would be out there alone, so I asked my friend Dennis to come and pace me on my last loop. The course had two steep hills and one hill was a half mile. My second loop was very scary and I heard a pack of wolves howling so loud I got scared and contemplated in dropping out. I finished at 2am in 7:28:28.

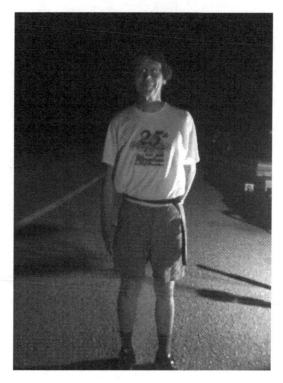

Dennis at the Cool Moon 12 Hour Run

In keeping my momentum up, I scheduled a double in the beautiful San Francisco Bay Area. I love the Bay Area! I'm from there and took all of its beauty for granted. I never really explored it until I started marathons. I have done Sequoia Trail Run 50K marathon number sixty-three many times and its one of my favorite trails. I'm feeling great and the weather is perfect. The course travels through the beautiful Joaquin Miller Park, to Redwood Regional Park with spectacular views of the Oakland Hills and the Bay Area along the way. I finished in 8:17:38.

Marathon sixty-four was the San Francisco Marathon. I met Marathon Maniacs from all over the country. The best part about the SF marathon is crossing the famous Golden Gate Bridge.

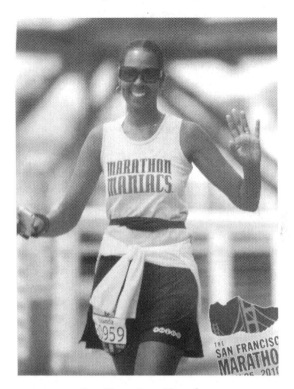

San Francisco Marathon

I traveled back to So Cal and participated in the Run the Beach Marathon. You actually get to run on the scenic bike path in Huntington Beach, California, I finished in 6:46:48.

CHAPTER TEN

AUGUST 2010

After Run the Beach Marathon I headed to marathon number sixty-six the Skyline 50K. I really like this race it's challenging, brutal and scenic all in one. The finishers get a nice shirt, tote bag and a wine glass. The post race BBQ feast is awesome. I finished in 8:08:33.

Mt. Disappointment 50K lived up to its name. I have done many 50K's but this one had to be the most brutal. Mt. Disappointment challenged my endurance. The course was run on the finest trails and canyons of the San Gabriel Mountains which were incredibly scenic yet very strenuous and challenging. We had panoramic views of seven peaks, we crossed waterbeds, climbed over large trees and there were many single tracks. The course had 6175 feet of elevation gain and the last four miles was brutal, the altitude was not my friend. I finished in 9:16:40.

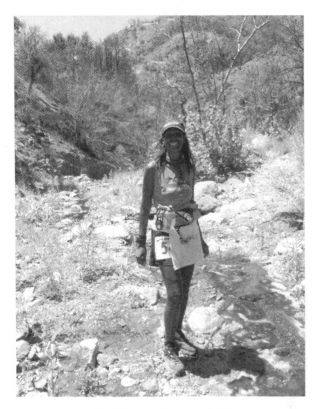

Mt. Disappointment 50K

Rockin the Coto Trail, I have done many times and it's also one of the scariest with snakes and mountain lions. I finished in 7:11:00. The Cinderella Trail Marathon number sixty-nine is also a trail I have done many times. The race director changed the course and I kept getting confused on the trail. I managed to pull it together in the end and completed the trail in 7:45:00.

After finishing the Cinderella Trail Marathon, I drove 250 miles on the scenic Highway 101to Los Osos, California for Montana de Ore Trail 50K. The course features seven miles of shoreline, rugged cliffs, sandy beaches, streams, canyon, hills and a 1,347 foot climb to Valencia Peak Summit. There is a nine hour cutoff and a four hour cutoff at the first 25K loop. Climbing to the summit the second time was very difficult, and exhausting. I finished my seventieth marathon/ultra in 8:45:41.

Park City Marathon had a mandatory early start for walkers and slow runners which I was fine with. Park City Marathon's aim this year was to showcase the beautiful areas of Park City, Utah. The course was scenic with rolling hills, surrounding mountains, beautiful trails and paved bike paths. This was my third year and my best. I didn't get altitude sickness and beat my last year time by four minutes. I finished in 6:14:52 and flew from Salt Lake City to Las Vegas for the ET Midnight Marathon number seventy-two. I love the ET Marathon. The marathon is run on Highway 51 (375) in Rachel, Nevada, which has an overwhelming number of reported UFO sightings. In 1996 the federal government officially named Highway 375 the "Extraterrestrial Highway." I finished in 6:52:47.

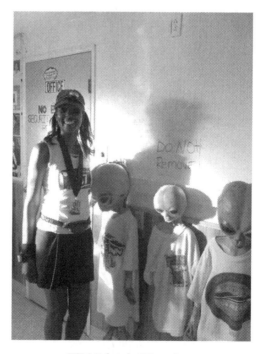

ET Midnight Marathon

Marathon seventy-three was a single marathon weekend. I was able to get some much needed rest. The Santa Rosa Marathon was held in Santa Rosa, CA. The course was scenic and beautiful and we crossed bridges, vineyards, cornfields, horse ranches and creeks. They had lovely finisher's medals and shirts and I finished in 6:12:05. I completed eight marathons in the month of August.

CHAPTER ELEVEN

AMAZING RACE

The next four races I called my own "Amazing Race". I did a quad, four marathons in four states in three days! I was both nervous and excited at what I was mentally and physically about to endure. I flew out of LAX to Salt Lake City and rented a car and drove 2.5 hours to Pocatello, Idaho for the Pocatello Marathon on September fourth. I like Pocatello's small town marathon with the big city feel. I finished in 5:58:41 and headed back to Salt Lake City Airport.

My flight out of Salt Lake City was on time and I arrived in Phoenix around 5pm. My son, who lived in the area, picked me up and drove me to Buckeye for the Buckeye Marathon. The marathon didn't start until 8pm but I asked the race director if I could start early. He told me no but if you changed my entry from a marathon to a 100K I could start immediately. I paid the difference and started with the 100K runners. Buckeye Endurance Run was on a five hundred meter dirt track which was at the beautiful Nardini Manor Track in Buckeye, Arizona. I finished in 7:22:08. I managed to get a few hours of sleep and arrived home to shower for day two, marathon three, state three. Run the Marina Marathon number seventy-six, was held in Long Beach, California. The course was run along the marina and the weather was perfect, cool and cloudy. I quickly finished and headed to LAX.

My flight out of LAX to Denver was delayed and required attention from the fire department. We were on the runway for an hour or so and after two attempts to fly, we were put on another plane. I wasn't concerned about my life but losing a marathon. Day three, I arrived in Denver around midnight and had a two hour drive to Colorado Springs. I was extremely tired and sleepy. I checked into the hotel and only got an hour of sleep. I was so miserable and grumpy. The American Discovery Trail Marathon was part road and trail which was scenic and beautiful. I finished in 6:15:36. I completed four marathons, in four states, in three days. What an amazing race!

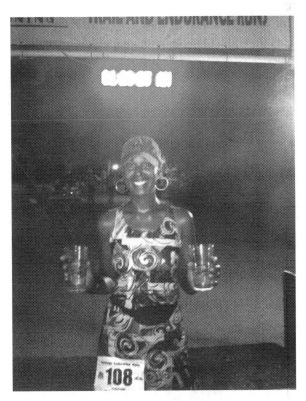

Buckeye Marathon

CHAPTER TWELVE

SEPTEMBER 2010

The Endure the Bear Trail Run, in Big Bear Lake, California started off as expected. I was having a wonderful morning until I received a devastating call from my niece. She called and said my eldest brother James, was in the hospital and I needed to get to him now! By mile twenty-five James passed from a massive heart attack, he was only sixty-two. I finished in 9:37:16.

I had to make a big decision on September 18, 2010. I was scheduled to participate in the Redwood Park 50K marathon in Oakland, California. That was also the day of my late brother James funeral. I made the painstaking decision not to attend his funeral. I know my brother would have wanted me to continue on my journey to Guinness. My husband attended the funeral while I did the 50K. I finished in 8:22:26.

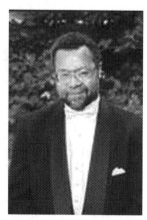

James Hampton

The Lake Tahoe Triple Marathons was my fourth and my best year. The triple covers the entire shoreline of the lake over three days. Day one of the triple I finished in 6:56:54. Day two was a beautiful postcard morning and I did a personal best in 5:59:33.

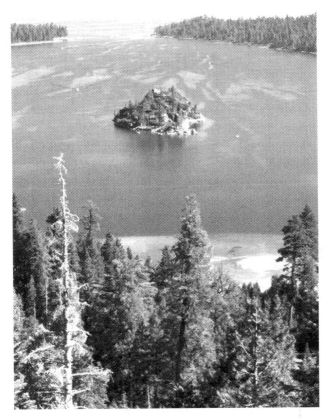

Lake Tahoe Triple

Day three of the Lake Tahoe triple was awesome and I had no altitude sickness, stomach issues, or headaches, just big fun! I finished in 6:36:3.

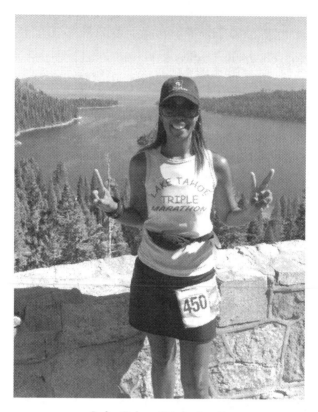

Lake Tahoe Triple day 3

CHAPTER THIRTEEN

OCTOBER 2010

The Camarillo Marathon was held in Camarillo, California and is a 1.5 hour drive from my home. Camarillo Marathon was an inaugural event which had a lot of issues. The weather was a cool sixty—four degrees and overcast. This was perfect for me after coming from Las Vegas the day before where I did not finish(DNF) at the Desert Dash Trail 50K. I got heat exhaustion at mile fourteen and had to quit. I finished the Camarillo Marathon in 6:24:09.

The Golden Hills Trail Marathon number eighty-five started in Berkeley, California at Berkeley's Tiden Park and finished 26.2 miles at Lake Chabot in Castro Valley. The course ran along the East Bay Skyline National Trail, which included fire roads and single track trails that provided gorgeous views of San Francisco, Mt. Diablo and the golden hills of the East Bay. I finished in 7:43:08

Wine Country Marathon was held in the beautiful Sonoma County wine country. We started in historical downtown Healdsburg and ran through a residential area of old homes and quaint streets. I passed many vineyards and dozens of wineries. The course had rolling roads with breathtaking views of Dry Creek Valley and Alexander Valley. The finishers medal is a must have for your collection and I finished in 5:57:24.

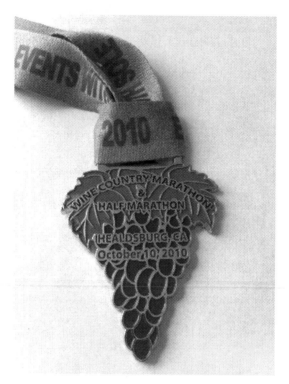

Wine Country Marathon Finisher's Medal

Marathon number eighty-seven was my third Mt. Diablo 50K this year and this time I was greeted by some creepy and scary looking tarantulas! It was mating season and the male tarantulas were everywhere. Just when I finally stopped screaming and tried to enjoy the beautiful scenery there was a stubborn rattle snake that wouldn't move. This caused me to finish my third brutal Mt. Diablo Trail 50K of the year a bit slow. I finished in 9:37:20.

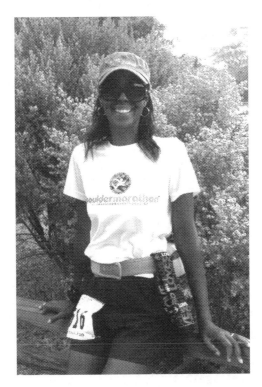

Mt. Diablo 50K

I finally completed my third California Dreamin series. The Long Beach Marathon was the most fun of all of my marathons. Nice course and great weather. I finished in 6:41:36 with only a few hours of sleep. I went on to do the Running with Sally Marathon in Lake Forest, California. It's on the Aliso Creek Bike path and the course was scenic and pleasant. I finished in 6:45:00.

I'm so close to my goal I can taste it! Malibu Canyon 50K was held at Malibu Creek State Park in Calabasas, California which is located in the Santa Monica Mountains. The park has beautiful views of the ocean, river crossings and amazing rock formations. I finished marathon number ninety in 8:04.

I had another fast weekend doing two marathons, in two states, in two days. I was ready for a sleepless weekend. The Hoover Dam

Marathon in Las Vegas started at Lake Mead beach and ran along the river mountain trail, the spectacular Mojave Desert, and through the historic railroad tunnel. I finished in 6:38:16 and headed back home to California. I couldn't sleep once I got home, so I decided to leave at 9pm and drive all night to my next marathon. My girlfriend Cheryl talked to me all night until I arrived in San Jose, California for the Silicon Valley Marathon number ninety-two. The course starts in downtown San Jose and makes its way through the heart of Willow Glen and funnels onto the Las Gatos Creek trail where I got attacked by Yellow Jackets! I got stung three times. I finished in 6:23:55 and finished off the month of October with nine marathons.

CHAPTER FOURTEEN

NOVEMBER 2010

I was so excited for race ninety-three, this was my first New York Marathon and what an experience. I was surrounded by forty-four thousand people from around the world all feeling the same excitement. It was a gorgeous ferry ride to Staten Island. I was very impressed with how organized the race was. We crossed many bridges, ran through Staten Island, Brooklyn, Queens, the Bronx, Manhattan, and ended in the world-famous Central Park. What a beautiful race day in New York City! The best part was having my daughter Tiffany waiting for me at the finish line. I finished 6:01:01.

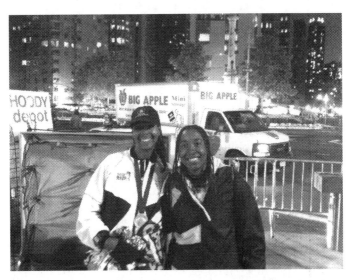

Tiffany and I at the New York Marathon

I got up at 3am to take the ferry to Catalina Island for the Catalina Eco Marathon. I got sea sickness on the ferry ride over. The course was hard and challenging with spectacular views of the Pacific Ocean. I finished in 7:09:59. I arrived early for the Malibu Marathon to pick up my race bib. I didn't get much sleep but was excited to do this race. The marathon is held in the beautiful city of Malibu, California home of "Two and a Half Men". The course was challenging, hilly and windy. I finished in 6:23:36.

The Mesquite Marathon number ninety-six was neither on my list nor in my plans. My advice to you . . . always have a plan B or race B! This advice I got from Mr. Larry Macon, Guinness World Record, "Most Marathons Run in a Calendar Year" by a man. Mesquite Marathon was not my scheduled marathon. I was scheduled to do Valley of the Fire Marathon in Overton, Nevada. After arriving to the Valley of the Fire Marathon, I was informed that the full marathon was cancelled due to gusty winds. I didn't panic. I remembered that there was a marathon sixty-four miles away. When I reached Mesquite the buses had left. I told one of the race officials my story and she immediately called the race director to arrange a ride for me to the start. I was only thirty-five minutes late, the race officials were my guardian angels that day and I finished in 6:43:11.

Santa Monica Mountains 50K was a beautiful morning in Malibu and a perfect day for an ultra marathon. The Santa Monica Mountains have an awesome view of the coast, inland grasslands and rugged mountain peaks. My journey was coming to an end and I decided to enjoy every moment. I finished in 8:52:34

There was a quadzilla (four marathons in four days) in Seattle Washington and I opted to do the triple. I traveled on Thanksgiving Day and spent three days in Seattle with my childhood best friend Cathy. The Wishbone Marathon, day one of the Seattle Turkey Triple was held in Gig Harbor, Washington. The race was run in Gig Harbor's beautiful Crescent Forest. The course was four loops around Crescent Forest; I did the fourth loop twice. Bummer! I finished in 7:45:00. The Ghost of Seattle Marathon, day two of the Seattle Turkey Triple was held in Seattle, Washington at Seward Park. The weather in Seattle was cold and depressing. I finished in 6:24:33. To complete my triple I completed the Seattle Marathon. I am now one marathon away from breaking the Guinness World Record for "Most Marathons Run in a Calendar Year" by a woman! I finished in 6:09:52.

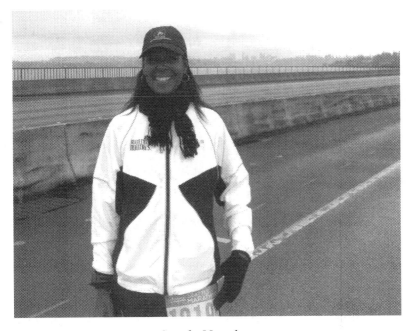

Seattle Marathon

Chapter Fifteen

DECEMBER 2010

The Rock N Roll Las Vegas Marathon in Las Vegas, Nevada was my record breaking race. It was December 5, 2010, and I had reached my goal of becoming the Guinness world Record holder for "Most marathons Run in a Calendar Year" by a woman! I was elated I had reached my goal and even more excited that I could finally rest. I am living proof that age has no bearing on accomplishing goals and expectations you set for your life. If you can dream it you can achieve it! I went on to complete five additional marathons and tied the overall world record with the male record holder, Larry Macon. On December 31, 2010 at the Savage Seven Marathon in Ocala, Florida, I ran a total of 106 marathons a great accomplishment but only the beginning! If You Dream It, You Can Achieve It!

I give thanks to God for giving me the strength and courage to take on such a huge challenge. God brings people into your life even if it's just for a moment. I could not have achieved my titles had it not been for all the love and support I received from my family, friends, associates and even strangers.

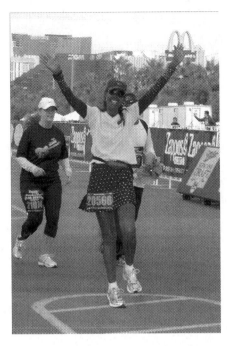

Rock N Roll Las Vegas Marathon

I stepped out of my comfort zone and with God's help, a little hard work, some motivation, and lots of determination; I was able to accomplish my dream. I gave myself permission to dream and envisioned the me that I wanted to be, and I became that woman. Yolanda Holder, loving wife, mother of two and Guinness World Record Holder! 2010 was a very exciting year for me. I held four titles:

- Guinness World Record, "Most Marathons Run in a Calendar Year" by a woman 106 marathons
- Marathon Maniac of the Year 2010
- Pacific Coast Trail Champion 2010 (age group)
- Blazing Trail Champion 2010 (age group)

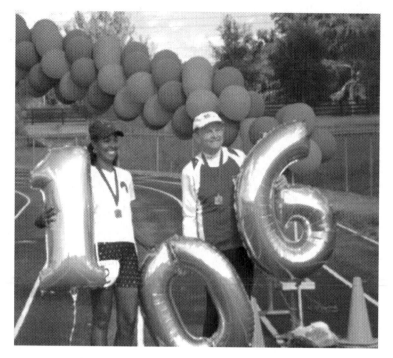

Larry and I at the Savage Seven Marathon

Marathon Listings & Completion Times

Texas Marathon, Kingwood, Texas/ 5:26:57

Kicking off the New Year Marathon, El Monte, California/ 6:55

Mississippi Blues Marathon, Jackson, Mississippi/ 6:02:51

First Light Marathon, Mobile Alabama/ 6:09:49

Museum of Aviation Marathon, Warner Robbins, Georgia/ 5:42:48

Rock N Roll Arizona, Phoenix, Arizona/ 5:49:05

Yuma Territorial Marathon, Yuma Arizona/ 5:40:33

Carlsbad Marathon, Carlsbad, California/ 5:56:16

Desert Classic Marathon, Goodyear, Arizona/ 5:57:17

Miracle Match Marathon, Waco, Texas/ 6:03:49

Diamond Valley Lake Marathon, Hemet, California/ 6:26:46

Surf City Marathon, Huntington Beach, California/ 5:37:43

Pemberton Trail 50K, Fountain Valley, Arizona/ 7:37:15

Lost Dutchman Marathon, Apache Junction, Arizona/ 5:58:41

Love your Heart Marathon, Huntington Beach, California/ 6:31:06.

Orange Curtain 50K, Cerritos, California/ 7:39:32

Pasadena Marathon, Pasadena, California/ 6:22:37

Cowtown Marathon, Ft. Worth, Texas/ 5:57:42

Mardi Gras Rock N Roll Marathon, New Orleans, Louisiana/ 6:04:35

Red Rock Canyon Marathon, Las Vegas, Nevada/ 6:03:53

Malibu Creek Trail 50k, Calabasas, California/ 8:23:38

Catalina Marathon, Avalon, California/ 6:12:28

Redwood Park Marathon, Oakland, California/ 6:38:47

Pirates Cove 50K, Sausalito, California/ 7:34:31

LA Marathon, Los Angeles, California/ 6:32:36

Napa Trail Marathon, Napa, California/ 5:32:58 which was a trail marathon PR!!!

Oakland Marathon, Oakland, California/ 6:08:30

Golden Gate Headland Marathon, Sausalito, California/ 5:30:07

Sycamore Canyon Trail 50K, Malibu, California/ 7:58:00

Labor of Love Marathon, Las Vegas, Nevada/ 6:07:51

Labor of Love 50 miler, Las Vegas, Nevada/ 14:10:36

Labor of Love 50K, Las Vegas, Nevada/ 8:41:02

Camp Pendleton Hard Corp Marathon, Oceanside, California/ 5:59:04

Skyline to the Sea Trail, Los Gatos, California/ 7:05:16

Rocky Road Run Marathon, Coto De Caza, California/ 6:11:10

Marin County Marathon, Marin County, California/ 5:52:50

May Day Madness Trail Marathon, Las Flores, California/6:39:15

OC Marathon, Irvine, California/ 5:45:40.

Quicksilver 50K, San Jose, California/ 8:07:48

Redwood Park 50K, Oakland, California/ 8:28:40

Palos Verdes Marathon, Palos Verdes, California/ 5:59:16

Going Bananas Marathon, El Monte, California/ 6:48:52

Rocky Horror Marathon, Coto de Caza, California/ 9:18:42

Hope Sight Mission, El Monte, California/ 6:49:58

Nanny Goat 12/24 Hour Run, Riverside, California

Memorial Day Weekend Marathon, Huntington Beach, California/ 7:29:09

Diablo Trail 50K, Clayton, California/ 9:58:11

Bear Lake Idaho, Garden City, Idaho/ 6:14:20

Bear Lake Marathon, Garden City Utah/ 6:11:09

Estes Park Marathon, Estes Park, Colorado/ 5:55:52

Angel Island Trail Run 50K, Tiburon, California/ 7:32

Father's Day Marathon, Coto de Caza, California/ 7:09:50

Five Cities Coastal Marathon, Oceanside, California/ 6:59:10

Running from the Devil, Lake Mead, Nevada/ 7:20:34

Running with Todd Marathon, El Monte, California/ 6:41:17

Stars and Stripes Marathon, Huntington Beach, California/ 6:18:50

Foot Traffic Flat Marathon, Sauvie Island, Oregon/ 6:07:07

Independence Day Marathon, El Monte, California/ 6:54:42

Dirty Dozen 12/6 Hour Endurance Run, Pinole, California/ 8:26:25

Sycamore Canyon Park Marathon, Riverside, California/ 7:21:40

Headland Marathon, Sausalito, California/ 7:15:25

Cool Moon 12 Hour Run, Cool, California/ 7:28:28

Sequoia Trail Run 50K, Oakland, California/ 8:17:38

San Francisco Marathon, San Francisco, California/ 6:20:52

Run the Beach Marathon, Huntington Beach, California/ 6:46:48

Skyline 50K, Castro Valley, California/ 8:08:33

Mt. Disappointment 50K, Los Angeles, California/ 9:16:40

Rockin the Coto Trail Marathon, Coto de Caza, California/ 7:11

Cinderella Trail Marathon, Oakland, California/ 7:45

Montana de Ore Trail 50K, Los Osos, California/ 8:45:41

Park City Marathon, Park City, Utah/ 6:14:52

ET Midnight Marathon, Rachel, Nevada/ 6:52

Santa Rosa Marathon, Santa Rosa, California/ 6:12:05

Pocatello Marathon, Pocatello, Idaho/ 5:58:41

Buckeye Marathon, Buckeye, Arizona/ 7:22:08

Run the Marina Marathon, Long Beach, California/ 7:12:00

American Discovery Trail Marathon, Colorado Springs, Colorado/ 6:15:36

Endure the Bear Trail Run 50K, Big Bear Lake, California/ 9:37:16

Redwood Park 50K, Oakland, California/ 8:22:26

Diablo Marathon, Clayton, California/ 8:31:36

Lake Tahoe Triple Day 1, Lake Tahoe, Nevada, 6:56:54

Lake Tahoe Triple Day 2, Lake Tahoe, California/ 5:59:33

Lake Tahoe Triple Day 3, Lake Tahoe, Nevada/ 6:36:33

Camarillo Marathon, Camarillo, California/ 6:24:09

Golden Hills Trail Marathon, Castro Valley, California/ 7:43:08

Wine Country Marathon, Healdsburg California/ 5:57:24

Diablo Trail Run 50K, Clayton, California/ 9:37:20

Long Beach Marathon, Long Beach, California/ 6:41:36

Running with Sally Marathon, Lake Forest, California/ 6:45

Malibu Canyon 50K, Calabasas, California/ 8:04

Hoover Dam Marathon, Las Vegas, Nevada/ 6:38:16

Silicon Valley Marathon, San Jose, California/ 6:23:55

New York Marathon, New York City, New York/ 6:01:01

Catalina Island Marathon, Avalon, California/ 7:08:59

Malibu Marathon, Malibu, California/ 6:23:36

Mesquite Marathon, Mesquite Nevada/ 6:43:11

Santa Monica Mountains 50K, Malibu, California/ 8:52:34

Wishbone Marathon, Gig Harbor, Washington/ 7:45

Ghost of Seattle Marathon, Seattle, Washington/ 6:24

Seattle Marathon, Seattle, Washington/ 6:09:52

Rock N Roll Las Vegas Marathon, Las Vegas, Nevada/ 5:59:26

Tucson Marathon, Tucson, Arizona/ 6:05:23

Rodeo Beach 50k, Sausalito, California/ 7:41:18

Zombie Runner Bay Trail Run Marathon, Palo Alto, California/ 6:41:53

Operation Jack Marathon, Manhattan, California/ 6:30:00

Savage Seven Marathon, Ocala, Florida/ 6:28:13

ABOUT THE AUTHOR

Yolanda Holder was born in San Mateo, California and currently resides in Corona, California. She has been married for 28 years to her husband Roger. She has two amazing children, her 28 year old son RJ and her daughter Tiffany, who is 26 years old.

As her children left the nest, she was relinquished of what she calls "the most fulfilling position", being a stay at home mom. She now enjoys spreading her message of getting fit and being healthy through motivational speaking and marathoning. Yolanda is among a group of women in their fifties redefining athleticism.

Her greatest accomplishment is being living proof that through God and perseverance you can cross the finish line! In her spare time she enjoys leisure walks, gardening, decorating and spending time with her family.

To learn more about Yolanda go to www.yolandaholder.com.